A COMPLETE DASH DIET COOKBOOK

50 HEALTHY RECIPES FOR WEIGHT LOSS

Table of Contents

Introduction

DASH stands for Dietary Approaches to Stop Hypertension. This type of diet is based on research carried out and funded on behalf of the US National Institute of Health (NIH). This research was about determining the role of diet on blood pressure. This diet was created to offer people who suffer from high blood pressure a delicious, tasty and balanced diet that lowers blood pressure at the same time. Therefore, this diet is primarily a diet to lower high blood pressure (more information on the DASH diet study in high blood pressure in the drug letter).

According to the NIH, the DASH diet promotes healthy eating habits. It offers healthy alternatives to junk food and processed foods. It aims to encourage people to reduce their salt consumption while increasing their calcium, magnesium, and potassium consumption.

Over the years, several other studies have proven the DASH diet is not only useful in lowering blood pressure, but that it is also useful in reducing the risk of cardiovascular disease, various cancers, stroke, diabetes, heart disease, kidney disease, heart failure and many more diseases.

The DASH diet is based on the following principles:

Reduction In Salt Consumption

One of the main goals of the DASH diet is to reduce the consumption of salt drastically.

Of course, man cannot live without salt. The human body contains around 150 to 300 grams of table salt. The amount of salt lost through sweating and other excretions must therefore be replaced. Salt supports the bone structure and digestion. It maintains the osmotic pressure in the vessels to keep the water and nutrient levels stable. But nowadays our foods are filled with too much salt - especially all processed products. The extent to which increased salt consumption hurts health is currently the subject of intense discussion among experts, mainly since the body excretes excess salt.

But studies from 1970 in Finland already show that too much salt causes blood pressure to skyrocket. It could be demonstrated that reducing consumption of salt by 30% could even reduce mortality from heart attacks by 80%.

A study on mice published in 2007 at the University Hospital in Heidelberg showed that a lot of salt increases blood pressure: "Salt promotes the formation of certain messenger substances in the muscles of blood vessels that cause the muscle cells to contract. The increased resistance in the blood vessels increases blood pressure." The Heidelberg scientists therefore saw considerable advantages in reducing the amount of salt in food rather than prescribing conventional drugs.

There is disagreement among scientists about how high the maximum amount of salt should be. While US experts recommend a maximum of 1.5 grams of salt per day, the German Nutrition Society's recommendation is 6 grams per day and the upper limit is 10 grams per day. However, this only applies to a healthy person who moves sufficiently and is physically active and excretes the salt again through sweating. For example, an athlete can tolerate more salt than someone who only moves moderately.

I recommend that you only look at these values as a rough guide and gradually control your salt consumption as well as gradually reduce it. Also keep in mind that the maximum amount of salt you should consume depends on your body constitution and lifestyle.

Recommendation:

- Less is more! Therefore, pay more attention to your salt consumption in the future and reduce it step by step. The keyword is low-salt, but not salt-free!

- Avoid processed products (packaged food, pizza, French fries, chips, canned food, various meat and fish products, baked goods, etc.). If necessary, read the list of ingredients.

- If possible, use a natural salt substitute (herbs, etc.) in your meals

- Use low-water cooking methods such as stewing or steaming. This means the food remains tastier and you don't need to salt it as much (see also tips on reducing salt consumption).

More Vitamin E And Minerals

The DASH diet is based on a variety of fruits and vegetables and whole grain products to provide the body with plenty of vitamins and minerals. Particular attention is paid to minerals such as magnesium and potassium, which help lower or improve blood pressure.

More Healthy Fats And Oils

Fats are energy carriers and ensure that fat-soluble vitamins such as vitamins E, D and K can be absorbed by the body at all. Certain fatty acids, such as omega-3 and omega-6 fatty acids, are also essential, which means we can only get them from food. Therefore, they should be on the regular meal plan. The omega 6/3 ratio plays a vital role in health. Omega-3 fatty acids help to maintain normal blood pressure levels wisely. However, our diet often contains too little omega-3 fatty acids. Good sources of this are fatty fish such as herring, mackerel, salmon, and sardines.

This also applies to the use of oils. Healthy oils include virgin cold-pressed olive oil and coconut oil (in organic quality versions). Unlike olive oil, coconut oil can also be heated and used for frying and baking. The much-used sunflower oil, on the other hand, is less healthy because it only contains omega-6 fatty acids. This creates an imbalance in the omega-3 to omega-6 ratio. A ratio between 1: 2 and 1:5 should be aimed for.

Ultimately, as with most other diets, the DASH diet should avoid unhealthy fats, especially trans fats, a subgroup of unsaturated fatty acids, and replace them with healthy fats such as those found in nuts, seeds and fish. Trans fatty acids come from industrial production and are, for example, contained in chips, baked goods, French fries, confectionery, pizza, etc.

More Fiber

Fiber is an integral part of the DASH diet. A fiber-rich diet, whether through fruits, vegetables, grains and cereals, has a positive effect on blood pressure and the cardiovascular system. (Evaluation of 24 publications between 1966-2003).

In contrast to the low carb diet, grain can therefore be consumed. However, it is essential to consume only wholesome grains (whole grain bread).

The diet helps in other ways. The foods included in the diet are rich in fiber, vitamins, and minerals. Potassium, magnesium, and calcium are necessary to control blood pressure, and are an essential component to DASH. When it comes to keeping cholesterol and blood sugar levels under control, fiber is particularly beneficial.

This is one of the ways DASH helps people to lose weight and in turn, by losing weight, you control your blood pressure. It is not uncommon for people using the DASH diet to lose up to 35 pounds in a few weeks without feeling hungry or deprived. Losing weight not only helps to control blood pressure but aids in preventing many diseases and ailments such as:

- Coronary heart disease

- Liver and gallbladder disease

- Colon, breast, and endometrial cancers

- Strokes

- Ulcers

- Skin infections

- Infertility

- Back pain

When following this diet, the protein and fiber from vegetables and fruit helps dieters to feel full. This is one of the best ways to lose weight without feeling hungry all the time.

Easy Ways to Make the Transition to the DASH Diet

Making the transition to the DASH diet is not as complicated as it sounds. Here are several tips that can help.

- Instead of water or tea with your meals, a glass of skim milk can be substituted. The milk increases protein and does not raise cholesterol levels.

- Keeping fresh vegetables and fruits handy can help by reducing the temptation to grab whatever can be found when hunger strikes. Instead of processed foods that are often loaded with sugar, healthy snacks are close at hand.

- When preparing meals; look at the labels. Canned food often is very high in sugar and sodium. Look for "no salt" or "very low salt" on the packages and labels. Check for saturated fats as well as sugar. This will become a habit in no time.

- If you use canned items such as tomatoes or beans, make sure you rinse them well before using. This will help to reduce the amount of sodium they contain.

- There are many dry spices that are quite flavorful, including cinnamon, paprika, and red pepper flakes. Mrs. Dash is a popular salt substitute and can be used to add flavor without the sodium. Did you know that ¼ teaspoon of salt contains 575 milligrams of sodium?

- Do you have favorite recipes that you feel you cannot live without? Replace ingredients that are not DASH compliant with acceptable substitutes. For example, if a recipe calls for sour cream, low-fat yogurt can be used. Another example, when a recipe calls for heavy cream, replace it with evaporated milk.

- If you absolutely must have sweets try and stick with low-fat or fat-free versions. Use the amount recommended by the DASH diet.

Another way you can make this transition smoother is to make a list of the foods you and your family commonly eat. You may want to write down your meals over several days. Compare these to the recommended foods on the DASH diet. This can help you to see what areas you need to change.

Recipes

Breakfast

1 Strawberry Sandwich

Preparation time: 10 minutes

Cooking time: 0 minutes

Servings: 4

Ingredients:

8 ounces low-fat cream cheese, soft

1 tablespoon stevia

1 teaspoon lemon zest, grated

4 whole wheat English muffins, halved and toasted

2 cups strawberries, sliced

Directions:

In your food processor, combine the cream cheese with the stevia and lemon zest and pulse well.

Spread 1 tablespoon of this mix on 1 muffin half and top with some of the sliced strawberries.

Repeat with the rest of the muffin halves and serve for breakfast. Enjoy!

Nutrition: calories 211, fat 3, fiber 4, carbs 8, protein 4

2 Apple Quinoa Muffins

Preparation time: 10 minutes

Cooking time: 35 minutes

Servings: 4

Ingredients:

½ cup natural, unsweetened applesauce

1 cup banana, peeled and mashed

1 cup quinoa

2 and ½ cups old-fashioned oats

½ cup almond milk

2 tablespoons stevia

1 teaspoon vanilla extract

1 cup water

Cooking spray

1 teaspoon cinnamon powder

1 apple, cored, peeled and chopped

Directions:

Put the water in a small pan, bring to a simmer over medium heat, add quinoa, cook for 15 minutes, fluff with a fork and transfer to a bowl.

Add all ingredients, stir, divide into a muffin pan greases with cooking spray, introduce in the oven and bake at 375 degrees F for 20 minutes.

Serve for breakfast.

Enjoy!

Nutrition: calories 200, fat 3, fiber 4, carbs 14, protein 7

3 Amazing Quinoa Hash Browns

Preparation time: 10 minutes

Cooking time: 25 minutes

Servings: 2

Ingredients:

1/3 cup quinoa

2/3 cup water

1 and ½ cups potato, peeled and grated

1 eggs

A pinch of black pepper

1 tablespoon olive oil

2 green onions, chopped

Directions:

Put the water in a small pan, bring to a simmer over medium heat, add quinoa, stir, cover, cook for 15 minutes and fluff with a fork.

IN a bowl, combine the quinoa with potato, egg, green onions and pepper and stir well.

Add quinoa hash browns, cook for 5 minutes on each side on a heated pan with the oil over medium-high heat, divide between 2 plates and serve for breakfast. Enjoy!

Nutrition: calories 191, fat 3, fiber 8, carbs 14, protein 7

4 Quinoa Breakfast Bars

Preparation time: 2 hours

Cooking time: 0 minutes

Servings: 6

Ingredients:

½ cup fat-free peanut butter

2 tablespoons coconut sugar

1 teaspoon vanilla extract

½ teaspoon cinnamon powder

1 cup quinoa flakes

1/3 cup coconut, flaked

2 tablespoons unsweetened chocolate chips

Directions:

In a large bowl, combine the peanut butter with sugar, vanilla, cinnamon, quinoa, coconut and chocolate chips, stir well, spread on the bottom of a lined baking sheet, press well, cut in 6 bars, keep in the fridge for 2 hours, divide between plates and serve.

Enjoy!

Nutrition: calories 182, fat 4, fiber 4, carbs 13, protein 11

5 Quinoa Quiche

Preparation time: 10 minutes

Cooking time: 45 minutes

Servings: 4

Ingredients:

1` cup quinoa, cooked

3 ounces spinach, chopped

1 cup fat-free ricotta cheese

3 eggs

1 and ½ teaspoons garlic powder

2/3 cup low-fat parmesan, grated

Directions:

In a bowl, combine the quinoa with the spinach, ricotta, eggs, garlic powder and parmesan, whisk well, pour into a lined pie pan, introduce in the oven and bake at 355 degrees F for 45 minutes.

Cool the quiche down, slice and serve for breakfast.

Enjoy!

Nutrition: calories 201, fat 2, fiber 4, carbs 12, protein 7

6 Quinoa Breakfast Parfaits

Preparation time: 10 minutes

Cooking time: 20 minutes

Servings: 4

Ingredients:

For the crumble:

1 tablespoon coconut oil, melted

½ cup rolled oats

2 teaspoons coconut sugar

1 tablespoon walnuts, chopped

1 teaspoon cinnamon powder

For the apple mix:

4 apples, cored, peeled and chopped

1 teaspoon vanilla extract

1 teaspoon cinnamon powder

1 tablespoon coconut sugar

2 tablespoons water

For the quinoa mix:

1 cup quinoa, cooked

1 teaspoon cinnamon powder

2 cups nonfat yogurt

Directions:

In a bowl, combine the coconut oil with the rolled water, 2 teaspoons coconut sugar, walnuts and 1 teaspoon cinnamon, stir, spread on a lined baking sheet, cook at 350 degrees F , bake for 10 minutes and leave aside to cool down.

In a small pan, combine the apples with the vanilla, 1 teaspoon cinnamon, 1 tablespoon coconut sugar and the water, stir, cook over medium heat for 10 minutes and take off heat.

In a bowl, combine the quinoa with 1 teaspoon cinnamon and 2 cups yogurt and stir.

Divide the quinoa mix into bowls, then divide the apple compote and top with the crumble mix.

Serve for breakfast.

Enjoy!

Nutrition: calories 188, fat 3, fiber 6, carbs 12, protein 7

7 Breakfast Quinoa Cakes

Preparation time: 10 minutes

Cooking time: 30 minutes

Servings: 4

Ingredients:

1 cup quinoa

2 cups cauliflower, chopped

1 and ½ cups chicken stock

½ cup low-fat cheddar, shredded

½ cup low-fat parmesan, grated

1 egg

A pinch of black pepper

2 tablespoons canola oil

Directions:

In a pot, combine the quinoa with the cauliflower, stock and pepper, stir, bring to a simmer over medium heat and cook for 20 minutes/

Add cheddar and the eggs, stir well, shape medium cakes out of this mix and dredge them in the parmesan.

Add the quinoa cakes. cook for 4-5 minutes on each side on a heated pan with the oil over medium-high heat, divide between plates and serve for breakfast. Enjoy!

Nutrition: calories 199, fat 3, fiber 4, carbs 8, carbs 14, protein 6

Soup

8 Vietnamese Beef Stew

Preparation Time: 15 minutes

Cooking Time: 8 hours

Servings: 6

Ingredients:

2 cups Beef Broth (here), or store bought

1 tablespoon cornstarch

1 pound stew beef, trimmed and cut into 1-inch cubes

3 carrots, peeled and chopped

1 onion, sliced

1 (14-ounce) can crushed tomatoes, with their juice

1 tablespoon honey

1 teaspoon Asian fish sauce

1 tablespoon five-spice powder

1 teaspoon garlic powder

1/4 teaspoons freshly ground black pepper

Directions:

In a small bowl, whisk together the broth and cornstarch.

Add the mixture to your slow cooker, along with the remaining ingredients.

Cover and cook on low for 8 hours.

Nutrition: Calories: 187; Total Fat: 5g; Saturated Fat: 0g; Cholesterol: 0mg; Carbohydrates: 15g; Fiber: 4g; Protein: 20g

9 Portuguese Kale and Sausage Soup

Preparation time: 10 minutes

Cooking Time: 35 minutes

Serving: 4

Ingredients:

1 yellow onion, chopped

16 ounces sausage, chopped

3 sweet potatoes, chopped

4 cups chicken stock

1 pound kale, chopped

pepper as needed

Directions:

Take a pot and place it over medium heat.

Add sausage and brown both sides.

Transfer to bowl.

Heat pot again over medium heat.

Add onion and stir for 5 minutes.

Add stock, sweet potatoes, stir and bring to a simmer.

Cook for 20 minutes.

Use an immersion blender to blend.

Add kale and pepper and simmer for 2 minutes over low heat.

Ladle soup to bowls and top with sausage with pieces.

Serve and enjoy!

Nutrition:

Calories: 200

Fat: 2g

Carbohydrates: 6g

Protein:8g

10   Dazzling Pizza Soup

Preparation time: 5 minutes

Cooking Time: 30 minutes

Serving: 6

Ingredients:

12 ounces chicken meat, sliced

4 ounces uncured pepperoni

1 can 25 ounces marinara

1 can 14.5 ounces fire roasted tomatoes

1 large onion, diced

15 ounces mushrooms, sliced

1 can 3 ounce sliced black olives

1 tablespoon dried oregano

1 teaspoon garlic powder

½ teaspoon salt

Directions:

Take large sized saucepan and add in the peperoni, chicken meat, marinara, onions, tomatoes, mushroom, oregano, olives, salt and garlic powder.

Cook the mixture for 30 minutes over medium level heat and soften the mushroom and onions.

Serve hot.

Nutrition:

Calories: 90

Fat: 2g

Carbohydrates: 17g

Protein: 3g

11   Mesmerizing Lentil Soup

Preparation time: 10 minutes

Cooking Time: 8 hours

Serving: 4

Ingredients:

1 pound dried lentils, soaked overnight and rinsed

3 carrots, peeled and chopped

1 celery stalk, chopped

1 onion, chopped

6 cups vegetables broth

1 ½ teaspoons garlic powder

1 teaspoon ground cumin

1 teaspoon smoked paprika

1 teaspoon dried thyme

¼ teaspoon liquid smoke

¼ teaspoon salt

¼ teaspoon ground pepper

Directions:

Add listed ingredients to Slow Cooker and stir well.

Place lid and cook for 8 hours on LOW.

Stir and serve.

Enjoy!

Nutrition:

Calories: 307

Fat: 1g

Carbohydrates: 56g

Protein: 20g

12   Organically Healthy Chicken Soup

Preparation time: 10 minutes

Cooking Time: 12-15 minutes

Serving: 4

Ingredients:

2 cans (14 ounces each) low sodium chicken broth

2 cups water

1 cup twisted spaghetti

¼ teaspoon pepper

3 cups mixed vegetables (such as broccoli, carrots etc.)

1 and ½ cups chicken, cooked and cubed

1 tablespoon fresh basil, snipped

¼ cup parmesan, finely shredded

Directions:

Take a Dutch Oven and add broth, water, pepper and bring the mixture to a boil.

Gently stir in pasta and wait until the mixture reaches boiling point again,

Lower down the heat and let the mixture simmer for 5 minutes (covered).

Remove lid and stir in the vegetables, return the mixture boil and lower down heat once again.

Cover and let it simmer over low heat for 5-8 minutes until the pasta and veggies and tender and cooked.

Stir in cooked chicken and garnish with basil.

Serve with a topping of parmesan.

Enjoy!

Nutrition:

Calories: 400

Fat: 9g

Carbohydrates: 37g

Protein: 45g

Poultry

13   Sweet Potato-Turkey Meatloaf

Preparation time: 15 minutes

Cooking time: 25 minutes

Servings: 4

Ingredients:

1 large sweet potato, peeled and cubed

1-pound ground turkey (breast)

1 large egg

1 small sweet onion, finely chopped

2 cloves garlic, minced

2 slices whole-wheat bread, crumbs

¼ cup honey barbecue sauce

¼ cup ketchup

2 Tablespoons Dijon Mustard

1 Tablespoon fresh ground pepper

½ Tablespoon salt

Directions:

Warm oven to 350 F. Grease a baking dish. In a large pot, boil a cup of lightly salted water, add the sweet potato. Cook until tender. Drain the water. Mash the potato.

Mix the honey barbecue sauce, ketchup, and Dijon mustard in a small bowl. Mix thoroughly. In a large bowl, mix the turkey and the egg. Add the sweet onion, garlic. Pour in the combined sauces. Add the bread crumbs. Season the mixture with salt and pepper.

Add the sweet potato. Combine thoroughly with your hands. If the mixture feels wet, add more bread crumbs. Shape the mixture into a loaf. Place in the loaf pan. Bake for 25 – 35 minutes until the meat is cooked through. Broil for 5 minutes. Slice and serve.

Nutrition: Calories - 133 Protein - 85g Carbohydrates - 50g Fat - 34g Sodium - 202mg

14   Oaxacan Chicken

Preparation time: 15 minutes

Cooking time: 28 minutes

Servings: 2

Ingredients:

1 4-ounce chicken breast, skinned and halved

½ cup uncooked long-grain rice

1 teaspoon of extra-virgin olive oil

½ cup low-sodium salsa

½ cup chicken stock, mixed with 2 Tablespoons water

¾ cup baby carrots

2 tablespoons green olives, pitted and chopped

2 Tablespoons dark raisins

½ teaspoon ground Cinnamon

2 Tablespoons fresh cilantro or parsley, coarsely chopped

Directions:

Warm oven to 350 F. In a large saucepan that can go in the oven, heat the olive oil. Add the rice. Sauté the rice until it begins to pop, approximately 2 minutes.

Add the salsa, baby carrots, green olives, dark raisins, halved chicken breast, chicken stock, and ground cinnamon. Bring the mix to a simmer, stir once.

Cover the mixture tightly, bake in the oven until the chicken stock has been completely absorbed, approximately 25 minutes. Sprinkle fresh cilantro or parsley, mix. Serve immediately.

Nutrition: Calories - 143 Protein - 102g Carbohydrates - 66g Fat - 18g Sodium - 97mg

15 Spicy Chicken with Minty Couscous

Preparation time: 15 minutes

Cooking time: 25 minutes

Servings: 2

Ingredients:

2 small chicken breasts, sliced

1 red chili pepper, finely chopped

1 garlic clove, crushed

ginger root, 2 cm long peeled and grated

1 teaspoon ground cumin

½ teaspoon turmeric

2 Tablespoons extra-virgin olive oil

1 pinch sea salt

¾ cup couscous

Small bunch mint leaves, finely chopped

2 lemons, grate the rind and juice them

Directions:

In a large bowl, place the chicken breast slices and chopped chili pepper. Sprinkle with the crushed garlic, ginger, cumin, turmeric, and a pinch of salt. Add the grated rind of both lemons and the juice from 1 lemon. Pour 1 tablespoon of the olive oil over the chicken, coat evenly.

Cover the dish with plastic and refrigerate within 1 hour. After 1 hour, coat a skillet with olive oil and fry the chicken. As the chicken is cooking, pour the couscous into a bowl and pour hot water over it, let it absorb the water (approximately 5 minutes).

Fluff the couscous. Add some chopped mint, the other tablespoon of olive oil, and juice from the second lemon. Top the couscous with the chicken. Garnish with chopped mint. Serve immediately.

Nutrition: Calories - 166 Protein - 106g Carbohydrates - 52g Sugars - 0.1g Fat - 17g Sodium - 108mg

16   Chicken, Pasta and Snow Peas

Preparation time: 15 minutes

Cooking time: 20 minutes

Servings: 2

Ingredients:

1-pound chicken breasts

2 ½ cups penne pasta

1 cup snow peas, trimmed and halved

1 teaspoon olive oil

1 standard jar Tomato and Basil pasta sauce

Fresh ground pepper

Directions:

In a medium frying pan, heat the olive oil. Flavor the chicken breasts with salt and pepper. Cook the chicken breasts until cooked through (approximately 5 – 7 minutes each side). Cook the pasta, as stated in the instruction of the package. Cook the snow peas with the pasta. Scoop 1 cup of the pasta water. Drain the pasta and peas, set aside.

Once the chicken is cooked, slice diagonally. Return back the chicken in the frying pan. Add the pasta sauce. If the mixture seems dry, add some of the pasta water to the desired consistency. Heat, then divide into bowls. Serve immediately.

Nutrition: Calories - 140 Protein - 34g Carbohydrates - 52g Fat - 17g Sodium - 118mg

17   Chicken with Noodles

Preparation time: 15 minutes

Cooking time: 30 minutes

Servings: 6

Ingredients:

4 chicken breasts, skinless, boneless

1-pound pasta (angel hair, or linguine, or ramen)

½ teaspoon sesame oil

1 Tablespoon canola oil

2 Tablespoons chili paste

1 onion, diced

2 garlic cloves, chopped coarsely

½ cup of soy sauce

½ medium cabbage, sliced

2 carrots, chopped coarsely

Directions:

Cook your pasta in a large pot. Mix the canola oil, sesame oil, and chili paste and heat for 25 seconds in a large pot. Add the onion, cook for 2 minutes. Put the garlic and fry within 20 seconds. Add the chicken, cook on each side 5 - 7 minutes, until cooked through.

Remove the mix from the pan, set aside. Add the cabbage, carrots, cook until the vegetables are tender. Pour everything back into the pan. Add the noodles. Pour in the soy sauce and combine thoroughly. Heat for 5 minutes. Serve immediately.

Nutrition: Calories - 110 Protein - 30g Carbohydrates - 32g Sugars - 0.1g Fat - 18g Sodium - 121mg

Seafood

18   Tuna Cakes

Preparation time: 10 minutes

Cooking time: 10 minutes

Servings: 12

Ingredients:

15 ounces canned tuna, drain well and flaked

3 eggs

½ teaspoon dill, dried

1 teaspoon parsley, dried

½ cup red onion, chopped

1 teaspoon garlic powder

A pinch of salt and black pepper

Olive oil for frying

Directions:

In a bowl, mix tuna with salt, pepper, dill, parsley, onion, garlic powder and eggs, stir and shape medium cakes out of this mix.

Heat up a pan with oil over medium-high heat, add tuna cakes, cook for 5 minutes on each side, divide between plates and serve with a side salad.

Enjoy!

Nutrition: calories 210, fat 2, fiber 2, carbs 6, protein 6

19   Spiced Cod Mix

Preparation time: 10 minutes

Cooking time: 25 minutes

Servings: 4

Ingredients:

4 cod fillets, skinless and boneless

½ teaspoon mustard seeds

A pinch of black pepper

2 green chilies, chopped

1 teaspoon ginger, grated

1 teaspoon curry powder

¼ teaspoon cumin, ground

4 tablespoons olive oil

1 teaspoon turmeric powder

1 red onion, chopped

¼ cup cilantro, chopped

1 and ½ cups coconut cream

3 garlic cloves, minced

Directions:

Heat up a pot with half of the oil over medium heat, add mustard seeds, ginger, onion and garlic, stir and cook for 5 minutes.

Add turmeric, curry powder, chilies and cumin, stir and cook for 5 minutes more.

Add coconut milk, salt and pepper, stir, bring to a boil and cook for 15 minutes.

Heat up another pan with the rest of the oil over medium heat, add fish, stir, cook for 3 minutes, add over the curry mix, also add cilantro, toss, cook for 5 minutes more, divide into bowls and serve.

Enjoy!

Nutrition: calories 200, fat 14, fiber 7, carbs 6, protein 9

20   Italian Shrimp

Preparation time: 10 minutes

Cooking time: 22 minutes

Servings: 4

Ingredients:

8 ounces mushrooms, chopped

1 asparagus bunch, cut into medium pieces

1 pound shrimp, peeled and deveined

Black pepper to the taste

2 tablespoons olive oil

2 teaspoons Italian seasoning

1 yellow onion, chopped

1 teaspoon red pepper flakes, crushed

1 cup low-fat parmesan cheese, grated

2 garlic cloves, minced

1 cup coconut cream

Directions:

Put water in a pot, bring to a boil over medium heat, add asparagus, steam for 2 minutes, transfer to a bowl with ice water, drain and put in a bowl.

Heat up a pan with the oil over medium heat, add onions and mushrooms, stir and cook for 7 minutes.

Add pepper flakes, Italian seasoning, black pepper and asparagus, stir and cook for 5 minutes more.

Add cream, shrimp, garlic and parmesan, toss, cook for 7 minutes, divide into bowls and serve.

Enjoy!

Nutrition: calories 225, fat 6, fiber 5, carbs 6, protein 8

21   Shrimp, Snow Peas and Bamboo Soup

Preparation time: 10 minutes

Cooking time: 10 minutes

Servings: 4

Ingredients:

4 scallions, chopped

1 and ½ tablespoons olive oil

1 teaspoon garlic, minced

8 cups low-sodium chicken stock

¼ cup coconut aminos

5 ounces canned bamboo shots, no-salt-added sliced

Black pepper to the taste

1 pound shrimp, peeled and deveined

½ pound snow peas

Directions:

Heat up a pot with the oil over medium heat, add scallions and ginger, stir and cook for 2 minutes.

Add coconut aminos, stock and black pepper, stir and bring to a boil.

Add shrimp, snow peas and bamboo shots, stir, cook for 5 minutes, ladle into bowls and serve.

Enjoy!

Nutrition: calories 200, fat 3, fiber 2, carbs 4, protein 14

Vegetarian and Vegan

22   Vegan Chili

Preparation time: 15 minutes

Cooking time: 25 minutes

Servings: 4

Ingredients:

½ cup bulgur

1 cup tomatoes, chopped

1 chili pepper, chopped

1 cup red kidney beans, cooked

2 cups low-sodium vegetable broth

1 teaspoon tomato paste

½ cup celery stalk, chopped

Directions:

1. Put all ingredients in the big saucepan and stir well. Close the lid and simmer the chili for 25 minutes over medium-low heat.

Nutrition: Calories 234 Protein 13.1g Carbohydrates 44.9g Fat 0.9g Sodium 92mg

23   Aromatic Whole Grain Spaghetti

Preparation time: 15 minutes

Cooking time: 10 minutes

Servings: 2

Ingredients:

1 teaspoon dried basil

¼ cup of soy milk

6 oz whole-grain spaghetti

2 cups of water

1 teaspoon ground nutmeg

Directions:

1. Bring the water to boil, add spaghetti, and cook them for 8-10 minutes. Meanwhile, bring the soy milk to boil. Drain the cooked spaghetti and mix them up with soy milk, ground nutmeg, and dried basil. Stir the meal well.

Nutrition: Calories 128 Protein 5.6g Carbohydrates 25g Fat 1.4g Sodium 25mg

24   Chunky Tomatoes

Preparation time: 15 minutes

Cooking time: 15 minutes

Servings: 3

Ingredients:

2 cups plum tomatoes, roughly chopped

½ cup onion, diced

½ teaspoon garlic, diced

1 teaspoon Italian seasonings

1 teaspoon canola oil

1 chili pepper, chopped

Directions:

1. Heat canola oil in the saucepan. Add chili pepper and onion. Cook the vegetables for 5 minutes. Stir them from time to time. After this, add tomatoes, garlic, and Italian seasonings. Close the lid and sauté the dish for 10 minutes.

Nutrition: Calories 550 Protein 1.7g Carbohydrates 8.4g Fat 2.3g Sodium 17mg

25   Baked Falafel

Preparation time: 15 minutes

Cooking time: 25 minutes

Servings: 6

Ingredients:

2 cups chickpeas, cooked

1 yellow onion, diced

3 tablespoons olive oil

1 cup fresh parsley, chopped

1 teaspoon ground cumin

½ teaspoon coriander

2 garlic cloves, diced

Directions:

1. Blend all fixing in the food processor. Preheat the oven to 375F. Then line the baking tray with the baking paper. Make the balls from the chickpeas mixture and press them gently in the shape of the falafel. Put the falafel in the tray and bake in the oven for 25 minutes.

Nutrition: Calories 316 Protein 13.5g Carbohydrates 43.3g Fat 11.2g Fiber 12.4g Sodium 23mg

26   Paella

Preparation time: 15 minutes

Cooking time: 25 minutes

Servings: 6

Ingredients:

1 teaspoon dried saffron

1 cup short-grain rice

1 tablespoon olive oil

2 cups of water

1 teaspoon chili flakes

6 oz artichoke hearts, chopped

½ cup green peas

1 onion, sliced

1 cup bell pepper, sliced

Directions:

1. Pour water into the saucepan. Add rice and cook it for 15 minutes. Meanwhile, heat olive oil in the skillet. Add dried saffron, chili flakes, onion, and bell pepper. Roast the vegetables for 5 minutes.

2. Add them to the cooked rice. Then add artichoke hearts and green peas. Stir the paella well and cook it for 10 minutes over low heat.

Nutrition: Calories 170 Protein 4.2g Carbohydrates 32.7g Fat 2.7g Sodium 33mg

27   Mushroom Cakes

Preparation time: 15 minutes

Cooking time: 10 minutes

Servings: 4

Ingredients:

2 cups mushrooms, chopped

3 garlic cloves, chopped

1 tablespoon dried dill

1 egg, beaten

¼ cup of rice, cooked

1 tablespoon sesame oil

1 teaspoon chili powder

Directions:

1. Grind the mushrooms in the food processor. Add garlic, dill, egg, rice, and chili powder. Blend the mixture for 10 seconds. After this, heat sesame oil for 1 minute.

2. Make the medium size mushroom cakes and put in the hot sesame oil. Cook the mushroom cakes for 5 minutes per side on medium heat.

Nutrition: Calories 103 Protein 3.7g Carbohydrates 12g Fat 4.8g Sodium 27mg

Side Dishes, Salads & Appetizers

28   Green Side Salad

Preparation time: 10 minutes

Cooking time: 0 minutes

Servings: 4

Ingredients:

4 cups baby spinach leaves

1 cucumber, sliced

3 ounces broccoli florets

3 ounces green beans, blanched and halved

¾ cup edamame, shelled

1 and ½ cups green grapes, halved

1 cup orange juice

¼ cup olive oil

1 tablespoon cider vinegar

2 tablespoons parsley, chopped

2 teaspoons mustard

A pinch of black pepper

Directions:

In a salad bowl, combine the baby spinach with cucumber, broccoli, green beans, edamame and grapes and toss.

Add orange juice, olive oil, vinegar, parsley, mustard and black pepper, toss well, divide between plates and serve as a side dish.

Enjoy!

Nutrition: calories 117, fat 4, fiber 5, carbs 14, protein 4

29 Herbed Baked Zucchini

Preparation time: 10 minutes

Cooking time: 20 minutes

Servings: 4

Ingredients:

4 zucchinis, quartered lengthwise

½ teaspoon thyme, dried

½ teaspoon oregano, dried

½ cup low-fat parmesan, grated

½ teaspoon basil, dried

¼ teaspoon garlic powder

2 tablespoons olive oil

2 tablespoons parsley, chopped

A pinch of black pepper

Directions:

Arrange zucchini pieces on a lined baking sheet, add thyme, oregano, basil, garlic powder, oil, parsley and black pepper and toss well.

Sprinkle parmesan on top, introduce in the oven and bake at 350 degrees F for 20 minutes.

Divide between plates and serve as a side dish.

Enjoy!

Nutrition: calories 198, fat 4, fiber 4, carbs 14, protein 5

30   Baked Mushrooms

Preparation time: 10 minutes

Cooking time: 15 minutes

Servings: 4

Ingredients:

1 and ½ pounds white mushrooms, sliced

¼ cup lemon juice

3 tablespoons olive oil

Zest of 1 lemon, grated

3 garlic cloves, minced

2 teaspoons thyme, dried

¼ cup low-fat parmesan, grated

A pinch of salt and black pepper

Directions:

In a bowl, combine the mushrooms with the lemon juice, oil, lemon zest, garlic, thyme, parmesan, salt and pepper, toss, spread on a lined baking sheet, introduce in the oven at 375 degrees F for 15 minutes, divide between plates and serve as a side dish.

Enjoy!

Nutrition: calories 164, fat 12, fiber 3, carbs 10, protein 7

31 Garlic Potatoes with Thyme

Preparation time: 10 minutes

Cooking time: 30 minutes

Servings: 6

Ingredients:

3 pounds red potatoes, halved

4 garlic cloves, minced

2 tablespoons olive oil

1 teaspoon thyme, dried

½ teaspoon basil, dried

1/3 cup low-fat parmesan, grated

2 tablespoons low-fat butter, melted

2 tablespoons parsley, chopped

Black pepper to the taste

Directions:

In a roasting pan, combine the red potatoes with garlic, oil, thyme, basil, parmesan, butter and black pepper, toss, introduce in the oven and cook at 400 degrees F for 30 minutes.

Add parsley, toss, divide between plates and serve as a side dish.

Enjoy!

Nutrition: calories 251, fat 12, fiber 4, carbs 13, protein 6

32   Corn Pudding

Preparation time: 10 minutes

Cooking time: 15 minutes

Servings: 4

Ingredients:

8 ears corn, grated

3 bacon slices, chopped

1 yellow onion, chopped

½ cup coconut milk

½ cup basil, torn

A pinch of black pepper

½ teaspoon red pepper flakes

Directions:

Heat up a pan over medium-high heat, add bacon, stir and cook for 2 minutes.

Add corn, onion, black pepper and pepper flakes, stir and cook for 8 minutes.

Add milk and basil, stir and cook for 5 minutes more, divide between plates and serve as a side dish.

Enjoy!

Nutrition: calories 201, fat 3, fiber 5, carbs 14, protein 7

33   Corn Sauté with Bacon

Preparation time: 10 minutes

Cooking time: 12 minutes

Servings: 4

Ingredients:

4 cups corn

4 bacon slices, cut into strips

A pinch of red pepper flakes

3 scallions, chopped

A pinch of black pepper

Directions:

Heat up a pan over medium-high heat, add bacon, toss and cook for 5 minutes.

Add corn, pepper flakes, black pepper and scallions, toss, cook for 7 minutes more, divide between plates and serve as a side dish.

Enjoy!

Nutrition: calories 199, fat 3, fiber 6, carbs 13, protein 8

34   Pineapple Potato Salad

Preparation time: 10 minutes

Cooking time: 40 minutes

Servings: 4

Ingredients:

2 cups pineapple, peeled and cubed

4 sweet potatoes, cubed

1 tablespoon olive oil

¼ cup coconut, unsweetened and shredded

1/3 cup almonds, chopped

1 cup coconut cream

Directions:

Arrange sweet potatoes on a lined baking sheet, add the olive oil, introduce in the oven at 350 degrees F, roast for 40 minutes, put them in a salad bowl, add coconut, pineapple, almonds and cream, toss, divide between plates and serve as a side dish.

Enjoy!

Nutrition: calories 200, fat 4, fiber 3, carbs 7, protein 8

35   Coconut Sweet Potatoes with Thyme

Preparation time: 10 minutes

Cooking time: 1 hour

Servings: 4

Ingredients:

4 sweet potatoes, sliced

A drizzle of olive oil

A pinch of salt and black pepper

1 small thyme bunch, chopped

1/3 cup coconut cream

½ teaspoon parsley, chopped

1 tablespoon Dijon mustard

½ teaspoon garlic

Directions:

Arrange sweet potato slices on a lined baking sheet, sprinkle thyme, drizzle oil, season with a pinch of salt and black pepper, toss well, introduce in the oven at 400 degrees F and bake for about 1 hour.

Meanwhile, in a bowl, mix coconut cream with parsley, garlic and mustard and whisk well.

Arrange baked potatoes on plates, drizzle the mustard sauce all over and serve as a side dish.

Enjoy!

Nutrition: calories 237, fat 5, fiber 4, carbs 12, protein 9

36   Cashew and Coconut Sweet Potatoes with Thyme

Preparation time: 10 minutes

Cooking time: 1 hour

Servings: 4

Ingredients:

2 sweet potatoes, peeled and sliced

½ cup cashews, soaked for a couple of hours and drained

1 cup coconut milk

¼ teaspoon cinnamon powder

Directions:

In your food processor, mix cashews, milk and cinnamon and pulse.

Spread some of the potato slices in a greased baking pan and drizzle some of the cashews cream.

Repeat with the rest of the potatoes and cream, bake in the oven for 1 hour at 350 degrees F, divide between plates and serve as a side dish.

Enjoy!

Nutrition: calories 200, fat 5, fiber 3, carbs 9, protein 8

37   Sage Celery with Walnuts

Preparation time: 10 minutes

Cooking time: 10 minutes

Servings: 6

Ingredients:

2 tablespoons olive oil

5 celery ribs, chopped

1 yellow onion, chopped

1 teaspoon sage, dried

8 ounces walnuts, chopped

A pinch of black pepper

3 tablespoons sage, chopped

Directions:

Heat up a pan with the oil over medium heat, add celery and onion, stir and cook for 5 minutes.

Add dried sage, pepper, fresh sage and walnuts, stir, cook for 5 minutes more, divide between plates and serve as a side dish.

Enjoy!

Nutrition: calories 250, fat 7, fiber 5, carbs 9, protein 4

Dessert and Snacks

38   Banana Vanilla Cream Yogurt

Preparation time: 5 minutes

Cooking time: 0 minutes

Servings: 1

Ingredients:

1 medium banana

1 graham cracker

1 teaspoon fresh lemon juice

1 cup nonfat vanilla yogurt

Direction

Slice the banana into a bowl. Break the graham cracker into small pieces and add to the banana. Sprinkle with lemon juice and top with yogurt.

Nutrition 345 calories 4.3g fat 14g protein 63g carbohydrates 186mg sodium 201mg potassium

39   Baked Coconut Egg Custard

Preparation time: 5 minutes

Cooking time: 45 minutes

Servings: 4

Ingredients:

Canola oil spray

2 cups nonfat milk

1 cup unsweetened flaked coconut

4 eggs

¾ cup sugar

¼ cup melted unsalted butter

1 tablespoon vanilla

2 dashes nutmeg

Optional: sugar-free gingersnap cookies

Direction

Coat a nonstick 10-inch pie pan with canola oil spray.

Combine all ingredients in a blender and blend 1 minute.

Pour into pie pan and bake at 350°F (180°C) for 45 minutes, or until custard is set. If desired, top with a couple crushed cookies.

Nutrition 320 calories 18g fat 10g protein 29g carbohydrates 129mg sodium 157mg potassium

40   Fruit Potpourri

Preparation time: 10 minutes

Cooking time: 0 minutes

Servings: 2

Ingredients:

1 teaspoon lime zest, grated

1 teaspoon lime juice

6 ounces sugar-free and low fat lemon yogurt

1 banana, peeled and cut in 4 medium wedges

4 strawberries

1 kiwi, peeled and cut into quarters

4 red grapes

4 pineapple pieces

Directions:

Thread banana pieces, strawberries, grapes, pineapple chunks and grapes on skewers alternating them and arrange on a platter.

In a bowl, mix lemon yogurt with lime zest and lime juice, whisk well and keep in the fridge until you serve your fruit kebabs.

Nutrition: Calories 145, fat 2, fiber 4, carbs 34, protein 4

41   Citrus Fruit Salsa

Preparation time: 2 hours and 10 minutes

Cooking time: 12 minutes

Servings: 10

Ingredients:

1 tablespoon brown sugar

8 whole wheat tortillas, cut into medium pieces

½ tablespoon cinnamon powder

3 cups mixed apples with oranges and grapes

1 tablespoon agave nectar

2 tablespoon sugar free jam

2 tablespoons orange juice

Directions:

In a bowl, combine mixed fruits with agave nectar, jam and orange juice, toss well, cover and keep in the fridge for 2 hours.

Meanwhile, spread tortilla pieces on a lined baking sheet, sprinkle cinnamon powder and sugar all over them and bake in the oven at 350 degrees F for 12 minutes.

Divide fruits salsa into bowls and serve with tortilla chips on the side.

Nutrition: Calories 110, fat 2, fiber 2, carbs 20, protein 2

42   Pearl Asparagus

Preparation time: 4 weeks

Cooking time: 0 minutes

Servings: 6

Ingredients:

3 cups asparagus spears, trimmed and cut in halves

¼ cup pearl onions

¼ cup apple cider vinegar

1 dill spring

¼ cup white wine vinegar

2 cloves

1 cup water

3 garlic cloves, sliced

¼ teaspoon red pepper flakes

8 black peppercorns

6 coriander seeds

Directions:

Divide asparagus, onions, dill, cloves, garlic, pepper flakes, coriander and peppercorns into jars.

In a bowl, mix apple cider vinegar with wine vinegar and water and stir well.

Divide this into the jars as well, put the lid on and seal.

Keep jars in a cold place for 4 weeks before you serve it as a snack.

Nutrition: Calories 30, fat 0, fiber 2, carbs 4, protein 2

43   Shrimps Ceviche

Preparation time: 3 hours and 10 minutes

Cooking time: 6 minutes

Servings: 8

Ingredients:

¼ pound shrimp, peeled, deveined and chopped

Zest and juice of 2 limes

Zest and juice of 2 lemons

2 teaspoons cumin, ground

2 tablespoons olive oil

1 cup tomato, chopped

½ cup red onion, chopped

2 tablespoons garlic, minced

1 Serrano chili pepper, chopped

1 cup black beans, canned and drained

1 cup cucumber, chopped

¼ cup cilantro, chopped

Directions:

In a bowl, mix lime juice and lemon juice with shrimp, toss well, cover and keep in the fridge for 3 hours.

Heat up a pan with the oil over medium high heat, add shrimp and citrus juices, cook for 2 minutes on each side and transfereverything to a bowl.

Add lime and lemon zest, cumin, tomato, onion, garlic, chili pepper, cucumber, black beans and cilantro, toss well and serve with some tortilla chips on the side.

Nutrition: Calories 100, fat 3, fiber 2, carbs 10, protein 5

44   Hot Marinated Shrimp

Preparation time: 1 hour and 10 minutes

Cooking time: 2 minutes

Servings: 8

Ingredients:

2 tablespoons capers

½ cup lime juice

1 red onion, chopped

½ teaspoon chili powder

1 tablespoon mustard

½ cup rice vinegar

1 cup water

1 bay leaf

3 cloves

1 pound shrimp, peeled and deveined

Directions:

In a baking dish, mix capers with mustard, lime juice and chili and whisk well.

Put the water in a pot and heat up over medium heat.

Add cloves, bay leaf and vinegar, stir and bring to a boil.

Add shrimp, cook for 1 minute, drain and transfer shrimp to the baking dish.

Toss to coat well, cover and keep in the fridge for 1 hour.

Divide into bowls and serve.

Nutrition: Calories 50, fat 0, fiber 1, carbs 3, protein 12

45 Lemony Red Pepper Spread

Preparation time: 10 minutes

Cooking time: 0 minutes

Servings: 16

Ingredients:

1 cup red bell pepper, roasted and sliced

1 tablespoon olive oil

2 tablespoons white sesame seeds

2 cups canned chickpeas, drained

1 tablespoon lemon juice

1 teaspoon garlic powder

1 teaspoon onion powder

A pinch of sea salt

A pinch of cayenne pepper

1 and ¼ teaspoons cumin, ground

Directions:

In your food processor, mix red bell pepper with oil, sesame seeds, chickpeas, lemon juice, garlic and onion powder, salt, cayenne pepper and cumin and pulse really well.

Divide into serving bowls and serve cold.

Nutrition: Calories 50, fat 2, fiber 2, carbs 7, protein 3

46   Low-Fat Trout Spread

Preparation time: 10 minutes

Cooking time: 0 minutes

Servings: 12

Ingredients:

½ cup low fat cottage cheese

¼ pound smoked trout fillet, skinless and flaked

2 teaspoons lemon juice

¼ cup red onion, chopped

1 teaspoon chili powder

1 celery stick, chopped

½ teaspoon apple vinegar

Directions:

In your food processor, mix trout with cheese, lemon juice, onion, chili, celery and vinegar and blend well.

Transfer to a bowl and keep in the fridge until you serve it.

Nutrition: Calories 40, fat 1, fiber 0, carbs 1, protein 5

47   Garlicky White Bean Dip

Preparation time: 10 minutes

Cooking time: 0 minutes

Servings: 8

Ingredients:

15 ounces canned white beans, drained

2 tablespoons olive oil

8 garlic cloves, roasted in the oven at 350 degrees F for 40 minutes

2 tablespoons lemon juice

Directions:

In your food processor, mix beans with oil, garlic and lemon juice and blendwell.

Divide into bowls and serve this dip with red bell pepper strips on the side.

Nutrition: Calories 89, fat 4, fiber 3, carbs 7, protein 2

48   Spinach and Mint Dip

Preparation time: 20 minutes

Cooking time: 0 minutes

Servings: 4

Ingredients:

1 bunch spinach leaves, roughly chopped

1 scallion, sliced

2 tablespoons mint leaves, chopped

¾ cup low fat sour cream

Black pepper to the taste

Directions:

Put spinach in boiling water over medium heat, cook for 20 seconds, rinse and drain well, chop finely and put in a bowl. Add sour cream, scallion, pepper to the taste and of course, the mint, stir well, leave aside for 15 minutes and then serve with pita chips.

Nutrition: Calories 140, fat 3, fiber 3, carbs 6, protein 5

49 Cilantro Spread

Preparation time: 5 minutes

Cooking time: 0 minutes

Servings: 6

Ingredients:

2 bunches cilantro leaves

½ cup ginger, grated

3 tablespoons balsamic vinegar

½ cup avocado oil

2 tablespoons coconut aminos

Directions

In your blender, mix the cilantro with the ginger, vinegar, oil and aminos, pulse, divide into small cups and serve.

Enjoy!

Nutrition: Calories 178, fat 4, fiber 6, carbs 14, protein 6

50   Cheesy Broccoli Dip

Preparation time: 6 minutes

Cooking time: 0 minutes

Servings: 4

Ingredients:

14 ounces broccoli florets

1 cup low-fat cottage cheese

A pinch of cayenne pepper

Directions

In your blender, combine the broccoli with the cheese and pepper, pulse well, divide into small cups and serve as a party dip.

Enjoy!

Nutrition: Calories 215, fat 4, fiber 6, carbs 15, protein 7

Conclusion

Thank you for making it to the end. Initially, when the DASH diet was created, it was solely created to reduce and stop the spread of hypertension, but it was later discovered that people who adopted the DASH diet were able to lose their weight to a considerable and moderate level. The reason for this was because of what the DASH diet entails that has made it effective for weight loss. As we end this book, here are some tips on how you can make your DASH diet work: Remove processed and junk food from your refrigerator: With the DASH diet, it is required that processed and junk food is rid of in the refrigerator because this food contains a high level of calories and unhealthy fats. Replace the processed and junk foods with fresh fruits, vegetables, grains, and raw nuts. Throwing away the junks may seem too much to do; however, the best thing to do is refraining from buying them.

Prepare a grocery list: Before heading to the supermarket, ensure you have a list of the DASH diet food list to purchase. This is to help to refrain from what is not on the grocery list in respect to the DASH diet Prepare your meal whenever possible: No matter how sweet and healthy a meal prepared in the restaurant is, you don't know the combination of the ingredients, whether it is a detriment to your weight loss or not. It is therefore important to ensure you prepare your meal all by yourself most times and by so doing you can monitor what goes into your body regarding the DASH diet Stock your kitchen with DASH food: To avoid the temptation of eating foods that are detrimental to your weight loss, stock your kitchen with DASH food from time to time. By so doing, you get accustomed to the DASH diet Avoid eating unhealthy snacks: Do away with snacks with unhealthy seasonings rather than go for snacks like popcorn cooked in olive oil and seasoned with garlic.

Dash Diet has gained popularity in the past few years as it is beneficial in strengthening metabolism and controlling hypertension. Contrary to the popular belief that while following the dash diet, one gets to eat vegetarian foods while getting a balanced diet that includes fresh fruits, vegetables, nuts, low-fat dairy products, and whole grains. You do not have to cut down on meat; instead, you have to reduce sodium and fat content from your everyday diet.

The diet also has many health benefits as it helps reduce hypertension and obesity, lower osteoporosis, and prevent cancer. This well-balanced diet strengthens metabolism, which further helps in decomposing the fat deposits stored in the body. As a result, it improves and enhance the overall health of a person.

This cookbook has provided you different Dash meals from breakfast, lunch, dinner, mains, side dishes, fish and seafood, poultry, vegetables, soups, salads, snacks, and desserts. However, you can consult experts if you suffer from current health conditions or follow certain exercise routines, as this will help you customize the diet as per your requirement.

This diet is easy to follow as you get to everything but in a healthier fashion and limited quantity. Talking about the DASH diet outside the theory and more in practice reveals its efficiency as a diet. Besides excess research and experiments, the real reasons for people looking into this diet are its specific features. It gives the feeling of ease and convenience, making the users more comfortable with its rules and regulations. Here are the following reasons why the DASH Diet works amazingly:

Easy to Adopt: The broad range of options available under the DASH diet label makes it more flexible for all. It is the reason that people find it easier to switch to and harness its real health benefits. It makes adaptability easier for its users.

Promotes Exercise: It is most effective than all the other factors because not only does it focus on the food and its intake, but it also duly stresses daily exercises and routine physical activities. It is the reason that it produces quick, visible results.

All-Inclusive: With a few limitations, this diet has taken every food item into its fold with certain modifications. It rightly guides about the Dos and Don'ts of all the ingredients and prevents us from consuming those harmful to the body and its health.

A Well-Balanced Approach: One of its most significant advantages is that it maintains balance in our diet, in our routine, our caloric intake, and our nutrition.

Satisfactory Caloric Check: Every meal we plan on the DASH diet is pre-calculated in terms of calories. We can easily keep track of the daily caloric intake and consequently restrict them easily by cutting off certain food items.

Prohibits Bad Food: The DASH diet suggests using more organic and fresh food and discourages the use of processed food and junk items available in stores. So, it creates better eating habits in the users.

Focused on Prevention: Though it is proven to be a cure for many diseases, it is described as more of a preventive strategy.

Slow Yet Progressive Changes: The diet is not highly restrictive and accommodates gradual changes towards achieving the ultimate health goal. You can set up your daily, weekly, or even monthly targets at your convenience.

Long Term Effects: The DASH diet results are not just incredible, but they are also long-lasting. It is considered slow in progress, but the effects last longer.

Accelerates Metabolism: With its healthy approach to life, the DASH diet can activate our metabolism and boost it for better functioning of the body.

Does this all flatter your hearts out? Of course, it does! So, start cooking now, and let us all be healthier and happier.

Consume less sodium: Food like bread, baked food, breakfast cereals, condiments, sauce, and canned products contain a high level of sodium, and these must be taken the required level to avoid posing a danger to the bodyweight.

Checking of labels: Most people are victims of the act of not checking labels on food items purchased; thus, endangering their health. Check the labels of every food item in your kitchen and refrigerator and dispose of anything that has a high intake of sodium, sugar, white flour, saturated or trans fats.

Portion control and serving sizes: This involves eating a variety of food in the right proportion and getting the required amount of nutrients needed. Eating to get overfed is what most people do all for the sake of eating to one's satisfaction, with this simple act, most people don't know that obesity can be gotten this, thus with the DASH diet, individuals know the amount of food to be taken with regards to the normal body functioning system and thereby having a balanced body weight.

Avoid Sedentary habit: This is a lifestyle that involves little or no physical activities. Examples of sedentary lifestyles are sitting with the computer all day long, reading all day long, or watching television most hours of the day. This kind of habit is not encouraged in the DASH diet, thereby not leading to unnecessary weight gain — more of a reason why the DASH diet encourages physical exercises.

I hope you have learned something!